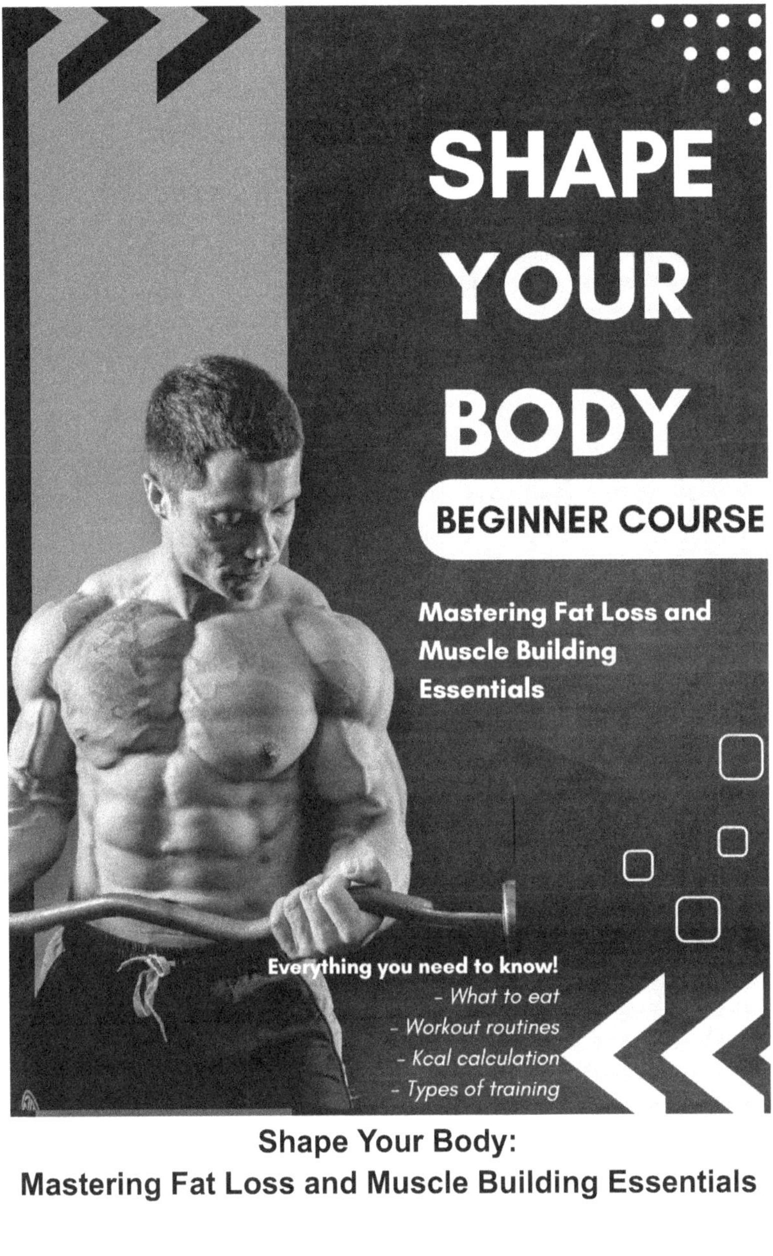

SHAPE YOUR BODY

BEGINNER COURSE

Mastering Fat Loss and Muscle Building Essentials

Everything you need to know!
- What to eat
- Workout routines
- Kcal calculation
- Types of training

Shape Your Body:
Mastering Fat Loss and Muscle Building Essentials

INDEX

INTRODUCTION..2

    CASE EXAMPLE:...3

IMPORTANCE OF TRAINING VS IMPORTANCE OF DIETING......................4

    Training without dieting:..4

    Dieting without training:..4

HEALTHY LIVE, HEALTHY MIND..5

BULKING VS CUTTING VS BODY RECOMPOSITION.............................5

    BULKING:..6

    CUTTING:..6

    BODY RECOMPOSITION (BEST OPTION FOR BEGINNERS 🏅)............7

HOW TO EAT..7

    - KCALS CALCULATION..8

    - PROTEIN - CARBS - FAT...8

    - DISH DISTRIBUTION (MAKE IT SIMPLE)...........................11

TRAINING FOR AESTHETICS VS STRENGTH....................................11

WORKOUT ROUTINES..12

    - AESTHETIC / MUSCULAR..12

    - STRENGTH / FUNCTIONAL...14

    3-DAY FULL BODY ROUTINE..16

CARDIO..18

    - WHEN TO DO CARDIO...18

    - TYPES OF CARDIO..18

    - RECOMMENDATIONS...18

SUPPLEMENTS...19

    - DO I NEED THEM?...19

    - IS PROTEIN POWDER HARMFUL?...................................19

INTRODUCTION

When it comes to achieving a good physique, most people think that they will need to sacrifice and suffer a lot in order to become who they want to be.

Some of them set unrealistic expectations such as losing all their body fat and becoming muscular in just a few months, and after not seeing big results in the first weeks, they give up and do not even keep trying.

Truth is that, if you are feeling that you are sacrificing too much and you are not enjoying the process, you are exceeding your limits and should adjust your training/diet to more achievable goals.

Having a good physique is not about destroying your body with super strict diets and hours of training, but it is more about **consistency**

CASE EXAMPLE:

- **Person A:** After living a sedentary lifestyle, decides to start a diet and join his nearest gym. As he wants fast results, bases his new diet into vegetables and chicken, quits all kinds of carbs and snacks, and starts training 3h a day, 5 times a week.

- **Person B:** Is tired of his body and decides to change his lifestyle, so he starts reducing the amount of calories in his diet by gradually removing snacks, junk food and sodas, to start replacing them with more quality food, making sure to not be hungry. Then, starts working out only 1h a day, 3 times a week.

WHO WILL HAVE MORE CHANCES TO ACHIEVE THE DESIRED PHYSIQUE?
While Person A set very strict requirements to achieve his physique faster, Person B understood that he will not be able to maintain such high expectations overtime, and decided to focus on the long-term goal

- **Future of Person A:** Burnout, since is eating too little and training too much, so his body will not have enough energy to recover. He might lose some weight, but as his lifestyle changed drastically, he was not able to keep the rhythm and ended up quitting thinking that it was too hard. ***As a result, ends up coming back to sedentarism and eating even more than before (due to this anxiety)***

- ***Future of Person B:*** Success. As his new lifestyle is not so different as he used to have, he was able to continue with this. After some time, he was able to adapt to this, and decided to make it harder, going 4 days a week instead of 3, trying to lift more weight, and reducing a little bit his kcal intake. **As a result, he adopted a new lifestyle, it is no longer hard for him to train and eat healthy, and he can keep improving without sacrificing too much.**

This teaches us that we need to set realistic and achievable goals, as we are planning to change our lifestyle in the long term.

If we plan to achieve a good physique fast, we will end up failing as we will not be able to maintain the rhythm overtime, and even if we achieve a decent physique this way, we will end up losing it as we will be starving to come back to our previous comfortable lifestyle.

IMPORTANCE OF TRAINING VS IMPORTANCE OF DIETING

Unfortunately, to achieve a lean and aesthetic physique, it is not enough to just start training, or just start moderating our kcal intake

Instead, we need to combine them, finding a balance between training and dieting

Results of:

Training without dieting:

- Outcome 1: If we are used to eating a lot and have too much fat in our body, we will gain muscle (as long as we are eating enough protein), but we will not lose too much fat. Instead, our body will end up looking even bigger and fatter, since our muscles will be hidden

- Outcome 2: If we do not eat too much and have a skinny body, we will develop a minimum amount of muscle, but will not be very noticeable. On the other hand, as a result of consuming our energy on the workouts, and not refilling them with enough food, we will always be super tired, and could become even skinnier than before

Dieting without training:

We will lose weight, but we will also lose our muscle mass. Therefore, we will not look lean and aesthetic, but small and flaccid.
If we lose our muscle mass, even if we reduce our body fat to low levels, our chest, belly, back and arms will not be defined

On the other hand, the less muscle mass, the less calories our body needs to maintain. Therefore, as we lose it, we will be needing even less calories than before, so our diet will need to be more strict than initially was.

HEALTHY LIVE, HEALTHY MIND

To achieve our goals, we need to understand that we cannot pass from playing videogames all day to training 3 hours a day eliminating all junk food from our diet.
If today you can lift 50lbs, will you be able to lift 250lb next week?
Of course not, that is why we need to change our lifestyle progressively
This is a change that is meant to stay in our lives, so it must be achievable to avoid the burnout effect.

If training 5 times a week is too much effort for you, you can start by training 4 or even 3 times a week, it is okay!
If you are used to eating junk food on a daily basis, you can start replacing some of them with more healthy, but yet tasty, options, it is okay!

Once we start getting used to it, we will see that it is no longer a challenge for us, and we will be able to step up and increase the level.

This change of lifestyle will not only have an impact in our bodies, but also in our minds
If you stay consistent, not only will your new good-looking body make you feel better, but also the feeling of having done what has to be done every single day will.

It is more than obvious that, most of people with aesthetic physiques display self-confidence, security, and sometimes strong personalities

This is the effect of success, they know they have earned that physique, nobody has given them that, it is their own effort and discipline what made it possible.

Needless to say, feeling like you have completed your daily tasks successfully, makes you feel better about yourself. This is what happens with training as well, your mind will be at peace after you finish your day. Having done what you intended to do.
With no regrets.

BULKING VS CUTTING VS BODY RECOMPOSITION

We all have different objectives, but when it comes to aesthetics, the type of workout we do in the gym will not mark as big of a difference as the diet.

To get into this topic, we need to understand that our body needs a certain amount of calories just to be maintained (for us to live), let's say, for example: 2000 kcals
- If we reduce the kcals intake from 2000, we will lose weight
- If we increase the kcals intake from 2000, we will gain weight

*We can see a more detailed guide about this in the **"HOW TO EAT"** part*

BULKING:

This is a phase in which we will be eating more calories than the ones we need to maintain our body.
The idea is to keep this process lean as possible, as if we get these calories out of junk food, we will not only gain muscle, but also a lot of fat.

For this, we need to be increasing the calories progressively over time. We can start by eating 100 more kcals a day. Then, after one month, we can increase it to +200 kcals a day

Once we get used to it, we can increase it a little bit more, but it is not recommended to have a caloric surplus of more than 500 kcal a day.

Lastly, remember that this is the **longest phase**. If you are able to maintain a **lean** volume, you will not be gaining too much fat, and most of the weight increase will be out of muscle

Then, you can keep the bulking phase for even a year or two.

Eventually, you will have gained some fat and you will not look as good as you wish, but in reality, you will have built a lot of muscle that is hiding behind that body fat,
Once you get there, it will be time to start your **cutting** phase.

CUTTING:

In this phase, your main objective is to lose body fat while you maintain the muscle you built.
It is not recommended to start cutting if you have not built muscle before.

As it happens with the bulking phase, it is best to reduce the kcal intake progressively, as if you cut a lot of calories in a short period of time, you will not only lose fat, but also muscle.

The cutting phase should be shorter than the bulking one. We are only here to lose fat, which can be done in 2-7 months

In this phase, we can start reducing the kcal intake by 300 calories, so if our body needs 2000 kcal to be maintained, we can start by taking 1700 calories a day.

Then, once we have lost some weight (1-2 months later, depending on the person), we can reduce it a little bit more, up to 500-700 kcals of deficit a day
It is not recommended to have a caloric deficit of more than 700 kcals a day.

BODY RECOMPOSITION (BEST OPTION FOR BEGINNERS )

If you are not used to doing physical exercise *(or have practiced sports that do not develop your muscles such as football, basketball, etc)* , have small muscle mass or simply have never gone to the gym, this is the best option for you.

Bulking and cutting is good when your body and muscles are used to the gym, but if you are a beginner, even if you do not have a high caloric surplus, you will gain muscle. And even if you do not have a high caloric deficit, you will still lose fat

As your muscles will not be used to the stimulus of the gym exercises, they will grow more easily at first
And as you are not used to burning calories out of exercise, you will lose fat more easily at first.

Therefore, the best option is to start consuming more protein, without having a big caloric surplus.

Example: Your body needs 2000 kcal a day to maintain > You decide to eat more protein, but always keeping these 2000 kcals, or even increase them a little bit to 2100 (can be done by increasing protein and reducing carbs/fats)

This way, you will **BUILD MUSCLE** and **BURN FAT** at the same time

But this will not last forever, eventually you will end up being stuck after some time as you become more advanced.

The results will depend on the person, you will need to be checking your own progress *(examples: daily/weekly mirror pictures, body measurements, etc)* and once you notice you are getting stuck, you can finish this process, but as an approximation, you can enjoy this beginner boost for a year at least.

HOW TO EAT

So we have explained how our bodies need a certain amount of kcals on a daily basis just to be maintained.
If we increase that kcal intake, we gain weight
If we reduce it, we lose weight

Then, let's see how we can calculate these calories.

- KCALS CALCULATION

You will gain or lose weight depending on the amount of kcals you are consuming compared to the amount of kcal you should be consuming to maintain your body

You will keep or lose your muscle mass depending on the amount of protein you consume

So we will be adjusting with the amount of calories to our goals, always trying to keep a high protein intake to avoid losing our muscle mass

To calculate your daily kcal intake, we recommend you to use online calculators.

We can just type in Google: *How many calories do I need* and will find some websites like: https://www.yazio.com/en/calorie-intake-calculator

On the other hand, you can use ChatGPT to calculate the amount of kcal you should be eating on a daily basis

Depending on your sex, age, size, weight and daily activity, you will need a certain amount of calories to maintain your body. Then, depending on your objective, you will need to add or reduce some calories from that maintaining amount.

Lastly, in order to calculate your kcal intake, you can also use **ChatGPT** to check every night, where you can describe your meals and ask for the total nutritional value of the day. That way, you will be aware of your progress, as you will be able to know if you achieved your daily goal or not

- PROTEIN - CARBS - FAT

While the amount of calories determines whether you gain or lose weight, the amount of protein determines whether you gain muscle (if you are eating enough calories), or you keep it (if you are in a caloric deficit to lose fat)

Protein is mandatory
- If you are in a caloric deficit and do not eat enough protein > You will lose muscle mass
- If you are in a caloric surplus and do not eat enough protein > You will gain fat, but not muscle

Now, ***how much protein do I need per day?***
The recommendation is 1-1.5g of protein per kg of body weight.
(1-1.5g of protein per 2,20 lbs of body weight)

Example: If my body weight is 70kg (154lb), I will be eating 70-100g of protein per day
More protein than that is unnecessary

MEAL	QUALITY
Fish	Good
Chicken	Good
Beef	Good
Turkey	Good
Legumes	Good
Striploin	Good
Tofu	Good
Eggs	Good
Peanut butter	High in kcal
Texturized soybeans	Good
Dairy (yogurts, milk, white cheese)	Good
Cheese	Greasy
Sausages	Decent
Hamburgers	Decent
Meatballs	Decent

Now, carbs are the meals with the higher amount of calories, so we will be adjusting our carb intake depending on our objective, to make sure we are meeting the right amount of kcals

Carbs = Sugar
But not all sugar is bad

MEALS WITH CARBS

MEAL	QUALITY
Rice	Good
Potato	Good
Pasta	Good
Fruit	Good
Cereals	High in sugar
Sweet potato	Good
Juices and soft drinks	Good
Corn	Good
Pastries	Good
Chocolate	High in kcal
Bread	Decent
Puff pastry	Good
Honey	Decent
Legumes	Good

The last thing to take into account are fats

Fats are not necessarily bad. In fact, they are necessary for our body
However, we need to distinguish between healthy/natural fats and saturated
fats
We need to be careful with saturated fats.

Normally, we will not pay that much attention to fats than we do with protein
and carbs, but it is good to be aware of how it works

The most important thing to take into account when consuming fats is to avoid
deep fried meals *(chips, french fries, fish and chips, breaded meats…)*

MEALS WITH FATS	
MEAL	**QUALITY**
Cheese	Saturated
White cheese	Good
Avocado	Good
Nuts	OK but low amounts
Dairy	Good
Sausages	Saturated
French fries	Saturated
Butter	Saturated
Cream	Decent
Bacon	Decent

Hamburgers	Decent
Homemade hamburgers with low oil	Good
Pate	Decent

- DISH DISTRIBUTION *(MAKE IT SIMPLE)*

If you are not willing to calculate your kcal intake, it is okay, you can make it simple too

If you want to be on a bulking phase:
- Bigger meals, as we want to eat more calories
- Half of the meal should be carbohydrates
- Second half of the meal should be protein
- Additionally, we should add some vegetables

If you want to be on a cutting phase:
- Try to avoid being full, it is better to eat multiple small meals than 2 big ones
- ¾ of the meal should be protein
- ¼ of the meal should be carbohydrates and vegetables

TRAINING FOR AESTHETICS VS STRENGTH

Firstly, we need to understand the most important principle of training:
Progressive overload
Every session, we should aim to increase the intensity of our training. It can be done by increasing the weight we lift, or just increasing the number of repetitions

Example: Last Monday, I did 100kgx4 reps in bench press, so today I will aim for 100kgx5

In order to be consistent with this, it is recommended to try to always do the exercises in the same order, as if one day we do bench press as the first exercise, and the next day we do it as the last exercise, fatigue will make a huge difference

TRAINING FOR STRENGTH:

In this kind of workout, we aim for explosivity, mobility and overall strength, so we will be more athletic with this type of training.

To do so, our routines will always have multi-articular exercises *(which are the most demanding)*
Such as squats, bench press, shoulder press, deadlift, rows… Basically, prioritizing free weights over machines

Then, as we are pushing our strength to the limits, we are not able to keep it for too long, so our rep ranges will be around 4-6 reps per set *(Example: 3 sets of 4-6 reps)*

TRAINING FOR AESTHETICS:

Here, we will aim for muscle growth for aesthetic purposes. Therefore, we will be focusing on recluting all those muscle fibers and isolating them as much as possible.

We will be using lighter weights with higher rep ranges, as we want to bring all the blood to the muscle we are working. Contrary to what happens when training for strength, we do not want other muscles to be involved here

For this, we will work more with machines and dumbbells, and our workouts will have longer rep ranges, being around 10-15 per set *(Example: 4 sets of 10-15 reps)*

WORKOUT ROUTINES

- AESTHETIC / MUSCULAR

1ST DAY (CHEST & TRICEPS)	
Exercise	**Number of sets x number of reps**
Incline dumbbell bench press	4 x 8-12
Incline chest flyes with cables	3 x 10-12
Flat chest machine / Bench press	4 x 8-12
Peck-deck	3 x 12-15
Overhead triceps extension (cable rope)	4 x 12-15
V-Bar cable triceps pushdown	4 x 12-15

2ND DAY (BACK & BICEPS)	
Exercise	**Number of sets x number of reps**
Chest row / barbell row (neutral grip)	4 x 8-12
Lat pulldown machine (wide grip)	4 x 8-12
Unilateral dumbbell row	3 x 6-8
Cable pullover (Z-bar or rope)	3 x 12-15
Standing dumbbell biceps curls	4 x 12-15
Scott bank curl	4 x 12-15

<table>
<tr><th colspan="2">3RD DAY (LEGS)</th></tr>
</table>

Exercise	Number of sets x number of reps
Barbell squats	4 x 6-8
Leg press machine	3 x 10-15
Romanian deadlift (dumbbells)	3 x 10-12
Quads extensions machine	4 x 12-15
Hamstring curl machine	4 x 12-15
Calf raises or machine	4 x 15-20
Hip thrust	3 x 8-12

<table>
<tr><th colspan="2">4TH DAY (SHOULDERS & CHEST)</th></tr>
</table>

Exercise	Number of sets x number of reps
Cable lateral raises	4 x 12-15
Dumbbell shoulder press / military press	3 x 6-8
Posterior delts machine or flyes	4 x 12-15
Dumbbell lateral raises	3 x 12-15
Dumbbell frontal raises	3 x 12-15
Flat or incline chest machine	4 x 8-12
Peck-deck / chest flyes machine	4 x 12-15

5TH DAY (ARMS)

Exercise	Number of sets x number of reps
Overhead triceps extension (cable rope)	4 x 8-12
Standing dumbbell biceps curls	4 x 8-12
V-Bar cable triceps pushdown	3 x 12-15
Scott bank curl	3 x 12-15
French press (dumbbells)	3 x 8-10
Pronated grip (forearms) Z-bar curls	4 x 12-15
ABS (crunches, plank, your preference)	4 x 12-15

1ST DAY (PUSH DAY)	
Exercise	**Number of sets x number of reps**
Barbell bench press	4 x 6-8
Incline bench press	4 x 6-8
Shoulder / military press	4 x 6-8
Dumbbell lateral raises	3 x 12-15
Overhead triceps extension (cable rope)	4 x 8-10
Body-weight dips / narrow grip bench press	4 x 6-8

2ND DAY (PULL DAY)	
Exercise	**Number of sets x number of reps**
Barbell row	4 x 6-8
Pull-ups	4 x failure
Chest row machine (wide grip)	4 x 6-8
Dumbbell pullovers	3 x 8-10
Standing dumbbell biceps curl	4 x 8-10
Scott bank dumbbell curl	4 x 6-8

3RD DAY (LEG DAY)	

Exercise	Number of sets x number of reps
Squats	4 x 6-8
Barbell deadlift	4 x 4-6
Leg press machine	4 x 8-10
Bulgarian squats	3 x 10-12
Hip thrust	4 x 8-10

4TH DAY (PUSH DAY)	

Exercise	Number of sets x number of reps
Barbell bench press	4 x 6-8
Incline bench press	4 x 6-8
Shoulder / military press	4 x 6-8
Dumbbell lateral raises	3 x 12-15
Overhead triceps extension (cable rope)	4 x 8-10
Body-weight dips / narrow grip bench press	4 x 6-8

5TH DAY (PULL DAY)	
Exercise	**Number of sets x number of reps**
Barbell row	4 x 6-8
Pull-ups	4 x failure
Chest row machine (wide grip)	4 x 6-8
Dumbbell pullovers	3 x 8-10
Standing dumbbell biceps curl	4 x 8-10
Scott bank dumbbell curl	4 x 6-8

3-DAY FULL BODY ROUTINE

1ST DAY (UPPER BODY)	
Exercise	**Number of sets x number of reps**
Barbell bench press	4 x 6-8
Incline bench press	4 x 8-12
Shoulder / military press	4 x 8-12
Barbell / machine Row	4 x 8-12
Lat pulldown (neutral grip)	4 x 8-10
Overhead triceps extension (cable rope)	4 x 12-15
Standing biceps curls (dumbbell)	4 x 12-15

2ND DAY (LOWER BODY & ABS)	
Exercise	**Number of sets x number of reps**
Squats	4 x 6-8
Barbell deadlift	4 x 4-6
Leg press machine	4 x 8-10
Bulgarian squats	3 x 10-12
Hip thrust	4 x 8-10
Abdominal crunch machine	4 x 12-15
Oblique crunches	4 x 12-15

<table>
<tr><th colspan="2" align="center">3RD DAY (UPPER BODY)</th></tr>
</table>

Exercise	**Number of sets x number of reps**
Dumbbell bench press	4 x 8-12
Incline bench press	4 x 8-12
Shoulder lateral raises	4 x 12-15
Barbell / machine Row	4 x 8-12
Lat pulldown (neutral grip)	4 x 8-10
Overhead triceps extension (cable rope)	4 x 12-15
Standing biceps curls (dumbbell)	4 x 12-15

CARDIO

- WHEN TO DO CARDIO

If our plan is to have an aesthetic physique, cardio is always a good option to help us maintain lower body fat percentages. However, we need to be careful with this

We should never base our trainings on cardio, and we should never start our trainings with cardio

We need our body full of energy for weight training, which will burn most of the carbs from our body.
Then, once finished the weight training, we can finish the session with some cardio

We can also do cardio on our rest days instead. This way we keep our body in constant activity, which may help our metabolism

- TYPES OF CARDIO

- **HIIT (**High-intensity interval training): This kind of cardio promises burning fat while resting after a very intense and short workout. You can search in YouTube: HIIT routine and follow the videos. *Normally takes 10-15 minutes*

- **Medium-high intensity cardio:** Running, boxing, rope jumping, swimming, bicycling, rowing machine, etc. This type of training is still very demanding and can take longer than HIIT training. *Can take 20-40 minutes*

- **Low intensity cardio:** Walking. This is the most underrated cardio, it takes longer but helps your metabolism and it is easy to complete as you can listen to music, talk with friends, use your phone number and even listen to podcasts while doing so. *8000-10000 steps per day is highly recommended*

As we are trying to build a routine in the long term to create a new lifestyle, we need things to be as simple as possible so that we don't get burnout

Therefore, high intensity trainings are, in our opinion, discarded. If you are not used to training, just going to the gym will be hard enough and you will need some time to adapt to it. If you do this kind of high intensity cardio too, you will definitely hate it and will not be able to keep it in the long term

Our recommendation is to find something that you enjoy
Normally, walking 8000-10000 is the most efficient and easy-to-follow method

However, if you practice a sport that you enjoy, keep it up! It is important to find the joy in our trainings, and most of sports can be considered as high intensity cardios, which will help a lot

SUPPLEMENTS

- DO I NEED THEM?

The short answer is no.

You can build an aesthetic and healthy physique without any supplements. However, some of them may help you a little bit with your progress

Supplements are meant to be taken when you lack something (e.g. omega 3 if you do not eat fish at all). However, with a balanced diet, you should not need any of them

Most supplements can help you in a very small percentage of your work. We can consider it a 0.10% boost

There is an exception, **protein powder**

You can refer to ***HOW TO EAT*** part in this course to see how many grams of protein will you need

As keeping a high amount of protein intake can be really difficult, specially if we are trying to cut and lose weight, protein powder can become our best friend here

However, we should never use it to replace any food. Our priority will always be real food, but if we are still struggling to reach the daily protein goal, we can use protein powder

There have always been several myths about protein powder. In the past, people used to see it as cheating; even comparing it to taking anabolic steroids

Nowadays, we have more information about this, as there are plenty of studies done about this supplement

Protein powder comes from milk serum, it does not have nothing to do with steroids, as it comes from a natural source

Protein powder will not affect our metabolism nor hormones

You can take the protein out of food or use protein powder instead. It will be the same

However, it is always recommended to prioritize real food and only use protein powder when unable to eat more / unable to meet your kcal&protein intake goals

www.ingramcontent.com/pod-product-compliance
Lightning Source LLC
Chambersburg PA
CBHW051932250726
48659CB00002B/967